MY STORY

I have experience of the condition, so am talking to you from the perspective of one who has suffered and dragged - crawled - walked through it all.

Here is my story:

Laying in bed one night watching Cirque du Soleil on DVD was a pretty normal night for me.

I would quite happily go to bed and put on a DVD and, like many, drift off to sleep very peacefully and comfortable.

What could be better than a nice sleep in a comfortable bed with not a second thought of anything else?

I remember the juggling act beginning then suddenly I began to breathe quickly and heavily and thought it was very strange.

My breath got shorter and my eyes began to go black as if I would pass out at any moment. Then the real panic set in.

The questions and intrusive, unwanted thoughts raced through my mind.

I had violent, horrific, uncontrollable thoughts that kept repeating like a broken record over and over and over.......

I began to sweat and gasp for breath not knowing what the heck was going on.

I stood on my feet but felt like I would fall over or needed to get on my hands and knees to stabilise myself.

As if I were vibrating!

My head felt dizzy and heavy, feeling like it was weighing me down, wanting me to slump forward and so I hunched over.

FIRSTLY A DEDICATION

TO LISA THE ONE WHO HAS BEEN THERE THROUGH IT ALL & BACK - THANK YOU FOR YOUR CONSTANT LOVE & SUPPORT.

TO MY FAMILY & FRIENDS (YOU KNOW WHO YOU ARE) WHO I AM SO GREATFUL FOR

TO MY DOGS WHO HAVE BEEN A CONSTANT SOURCE OF GOOD ENERGY

You will find my story in my other book too.

'There and Back, The Dark Journey': The Way Back From Anxiety, Depression and Pure 'O'

This book is an expansion of the one above and is one of my key tools.

I write so that I can help others who I cannot physically be with to become well again.

Don't give in, you will get there, keep pushing forward - the light will reveal itself again.

MAKE CHANGE BY IMPLEMENTING ACTION TO BRING ABOUT THAT CHANGE

I stumbled into my mother's room and she was really shocked to see me in this state.

Next, I slumped down onto the bed and began to cry uncontrollably into my hands - I just couldn't explain what was going on and I had never been as terrified in my life!!

Breathing was so difficult, as my throat seemed narrow and the air just wasn't getting into my system fast enough.

Constantly gasping for breath, I was in a whirlwind of fear, upset and pure panic.

It felt impossible to hold my head up and when I did, focussing through my tears was difficult.

I hesitated to tell her the intrusive thoughts that were in my mind as I thought she may think I was going mad.

We sat together for a while and she managed to calm me down; after thirty minutes of crying, I had literally exhausted myself.

Then we agreed that I should go back to bed, try to sleep and we would see how I felt and what we could do, which I did, but all I could do was lie awake in pure shock and couldn't believe or explain what had just happened.

I thought if I could sleep I would be ok in the morning and everything would simply be reset to normal.

After another few hours I managed to drift off to sleep, utterly exhausted.

As I woke, I still had the thoughts rushing through my mind and couldn't shake the feelings of fear and dread.

Hesitatingly, I walked into the kitchen for something to drink and I finally mustered up the courage to get some breakfast.

My mother was waiting for me in the lounge with a worried look on her face as she was as puzzled as me.

I couldn't contain myself as the breath began to become short again; my head spinning and I seemed to have trouble balancing my body.

Finding the courage, and out of pure fear and the need to know what on earth was happening to me, I confessed, with great hesitation, the intrusive thoughts and fears in my mind.

My thoughts were of a violent nature towards my family and pets, images of them coming to harm as if it were happening that very second.

I cannot begin to tell you how real these images seemed, they began to dominate my mind every second of my life, totally saturating my mind.

There was no escape, no gap for me to simply just chill out and relax, they were relentless!
As soon as one thought had died down another would pop in saying I was homosexual, which only set me off again with further confusion and disorientation.

All through the day my throat would close up as the onslaught of intrusive, unstoppable thoughts flooded my system.

The thoughts were of everything that I was not and would never be - my worst imaginable nightmares.

Immediately we scheduled an appointment at the doctor's surgery to see my local GP in search of answers.

Sitting there listening to the doctor didn't feel real; it was as if I was a ghost viewing the experience from above.

I felt numb and out of touch with reality; floating and simply watching from behind bars of what was going on.

Experiencing this sensation was upsetting.

I was trapped in a limbo like state numbed out from existence with only fear, anxiety and upset as my companions.

It was as if I had faded away and all I was able to do was panic, cry and be constantly frustrated, annoyed and disgusted with myself every second of every day.

Becoming numbed out of the ability to feel positive, joyful emotions and experiences became all too familiar.

This experience was again scary and made me worse and worse as the days turned into weeks and weeks into months and so on.

I panicked and just wanted to get home to sit in my room and calm down, simply trying to sort my head out.

The doctor prescribed me with the anti-depressant Fluoxetine, otherwise known as 'Prozac,' which I took religiously, praying it would restore a state of normality to my mind and life.

The feelings I had experienced were happening on a daily basis with regular outbreaks of crying, panicking and near blackouts.

I felt as though I wasn't breathing properly and couldn't cope with the simplest of tasks, such as walking into the garden.

I was so detached from everything and everyone, I couldn't bring myself to be physically near anyone.

When people attempted to hug me I felt repelled and my sex life - well, there was no sex life anymore.

Becoming more and more detached, distant and numb by the day.

We upped the dosage of the Fluoxetine to double strength in the hope that it would reduce the panic attacks and help calm my mind of these awful, vile, intrusive, unwanted thoughts and sensations.

It was as if I was in 'Groundhog Day' and didn't know how to get free.

The next step was counselling and then a round of hypnotherapy, then CBT and another set of hypnotherapy.

All of the practitioners tried to help me with their techniques but I had little to no success.

My quest to get better was becoming more and more discouraging by the day and I entered a deep, deep, deep state of self destruction and that's when I hit the bottom.

My thoughts had become of a suicidal nature at this point and were really upsetting; they made my throat close up and restrict my breathing, I was also crying more and more.

It was becoming a chore hiding the condition from my family - it took everything I had and left me crying my eyes out, I was in a constant state of exhaustion.

My father and brother were in the dark as I didn't want anyone else worrying and felt like they didn't need to be burdened with me.

I would regularly dash away from anyone, retreating to the safety of my room where I could hide from prying eyes.

I had lost my appetite and only ate when prompted to.

Yet again we tried the doctor and yet another anti-depressant in the hope a different medication would be the key.

I had really hit rock bottom and the suicidal, intrusive thoughts were relentless, it started to make me believe life wasn't worth this intolerable agony.

Having a total lack of faith in the doctor didn't help, although I knew he was just doing his job it really didn't help me simply by handing me pills and sending me on my way.

Not knowing what to do we decided to pay a specialist psychiatric doctor in the hopes he could at least give me a diagnosis.
At this point I would have done anything, I was getting really desperate and wanted to know what it was that had stolen my life.

I wanted my life back, so I thought if I knew exactly what this thing was, I would have a better chance of fighting it.

The not knowing is the worst thing in my opinion!

He advised another anti-depressant to take and then........

Pure shock hit me when I was diagnosed with anxiety, depression and wait for it.... OCD!!! Also known as, pure 'O'.

OCD!!!!!

Depression I knew and anxiety too, but OCD?

Unbelievable!!

I was in shock; in this dream like state.

I just didn't feel real and I had not felt a positive emotion in years.

Learning that OCD came in different forms, not simply checking and repeating things physically, but that there was a thought process side that many do not know or even consider to be part of OCD.

I later learned I had what many call Pure 'O' which is intrusive, repetitive, unwanted thoughts.

Crawling through life and simply surviving was no life at all especially in this state of self destruction and mental sabotage.

As you can imagine, I constantly searched online for a miracle cure to liberate me from my cage.

Every door seemed closed.

I remember one day where the panic and fear had totally taken over me I screamed and threw myself to the floor in a trance like state and cried my eyes out.
Feeling so frustrated and upset I punched the floor repeatedly with all my might.

Shaking uncontrollably we thought I would have to go to hospital; my mother had the phone in her hand but I said,

'No.'

This day was the worst I had had!

I felt like I was having a heart attack and going to die right there and then due to the sensations I was feeling.

I felt dizzy, sick, unreal, shaky, disorientated, floaty, out of breath, lump in my throat, throat closed, pain in my head, eyes and ears.

That is just what I remember, as it didn't feel real, I was so out of touch with my body and mind.

At this point I had given up all hope of ever getting well again.
My partner and mother basically helped me to hold on to my life in my darkest hours and I can't thank them enough.

I felt like a puppet and couldn't control the strings.

Having gone through so many scenarios from it being a mineral deficiency to being possessed by something, I just didn't know.

I just knew I could not go on much longer in this state.

At one point I considered seeing a priest to ask for his help.

After my research online, I found great solace in knowing there were others like myself who were having the same troubles and battling on as I was.

It was awful to know but there was an element of comfort, knowing I wasn't the only one.

Reading stories of people recovering gave me the speck of hope I needed to move up instead of down.

The internet had been my only reach to the outside world and my library of knowledge.

In addition to this I have many books on depression and have painstakingly read them all over and over in search of becoming well and 'Me' again.

Relying on a magical cure or formula just wasn't going to work and wasn't good enough.

After suffering for years I decided to take a different approach.

RESEARCH! RESEARCH! RESEARCH!

Thinking back now, having that small spark of hope in the darkness kept me going.

My partner and mother had kept me going, being like crutches under my arms, enabling me to simply exist until I realised the solution wasn't going to find me, I had to find it.

I stepped back and looked at my life as a whole and noticed big gaps where I was not fulfilling my body and mind's basic needs.

I used two keys to begin my recovery and I will talk about these later.

I do know how you feel and have experienced anxiety, pure O and depression myself for years.

So please keep the hope and have faith in yourself, there is a solution.

Suffering for years is horrid and having experienced it for myself I wanted to help others to get back up on their feet 'A.S.A.P' and begin to feel again and feel good.

Don't simply let doctors feed you pills, look outside the norm, keep the faith and be prepared to try anything.

I know for a fact that in my desperation I would have done anything to get back some quality of life and rid myself of the condition.

Literally anything was better than not living a ghostly existence of fear, pain and torment.

I have experienced treatments such as:

- Hypnotherapy
- CBT
- Exposure Response Prevention therapy
- CBT courses
- Counselling
- SSRI's
- Anti-depressants
- Natural relaxation remedies

The above were the only things I was able to try due to the fear of going out.

It took a lot more work for me to get my confidence and 'sea legs' back.

I have spent thousands of pounds in the search for wellbeing.

The condition can not only rob you of your drive and sanity but of your money too!

But as I keep saying, anything is better than the intolerable agony that I was suffering from.

I don't look at the money spent as money wasted, as I needed to go through what I had to, to be able to get to this point.

I can now function and am able to have fun which was an impossible task before.

Every aspect of my life has improved and I know yours will too but only if you let it.

Now I could go on and on but you have heard my story and progression to this point.

It's time for the ones who held me up through it all to speak and tell you their side.

My mother and partner have kindly agreed to write a little part to let you and your loved ones see it from their perspective.

It is really important to let others help you along your way and to help you recover, which you will.

USING NUTRITION AS A WAY TO COMBAT ANXIETY, DEPRESSION & PURE 'O'.

In today's society we are all victims of so many influential factors such as advertising and marketing of foods that have a negative response when ingested into our systems.

Gone are the days when our grandmothers and grandfathers used to thrive on the basic, bare minimal essentials.

I cannot describe just how much the world has changed in regards to nutrition and the evolution of the diet throughout time.

There are multiple books on diets and nutritional information that it can be very frustrating and difficult to know which direction to go in.

That's my reasoning for writing this book.

If you have read 'The Dark Journey' a book previously written by me you will know that diet was of paramount importance in my recovery of depression, anxiety and pure O.

I am a qualified personal trainer and nutritional specialist but my experience with food and diet goes beyond research and qualifications.

I have travelled the weight scales of time and as a result know what it is like to be at the high obese end of the scale and also at the low underweight end too.

So I can tell you my body has been through the experiences of weight gain and also weight loss.

Now you may think,' OK, so what's that got to do with depression, anxiety and pure 'O'????'

Well, diet is a vital component to gaining the advantage and overcoming these debilitating conditions.

Diet affects every function in the body and the foods we consume have a specific role when we eat them.

I cannot stress enough just how important your daily nutrition impacts on your health, wellbeing and vitality as well as your mental state and awareness.

We often overlook just how important it is due to our condition masking every element and experience of our lives.

When you are in the midst of panic, fear and dread, diet is the last thing on your mind.

So why write a nutrition book?

Well nutrition is the way of healing your body from the inside out.

It enables your body to function either at full capacity or to slow it down to a sluggish crawl.

So why not optimize your nutrition and gain the advantage on your condition?

I did and have the experience of creating a state of wellbeing and stability in my life AND STILL DO.

TAKE ACTION AND BUILD THE BODY AND FUTURE YOU WANT

WHERE DID THINGS GO WRONG?

I could go on and on about people consuming this, that and the other, but this book is not to reprimand you, it is to give my genuine knowledge and experience for you to either take onboard or to look in another direction.

THE CHOICE IS, AS ALWAYS, YOURS AS YOU HOLD THE KEY TO YOUR LIFE

If you do research on our diet through time you will notice that things have changed tremendously from wars, famine, greed, abundance, luxury, social climate, peer group influence, government recommendations, word of mouth and so on.

There are so many influential factors that seep their way into the news and mass media to the supermarkets and on the T.V.

All have such a massive impact on people and how they perceive things. We often just go on auto-pilot everyday and due to things like hectic jobs, family crisis, convenience, peer pressure, lack of time and knowledge, we get complacent and do everything for the ease of it.

As I say, I could go on but what I want to do is flip the switch and take you off auto-pilot and place the power back into your hands.

When we have the knowledge that we need to better ourselves, we can truly live to our potential and live with a body that will not only function better but will also thrive the way it should.

Once you give a body what it needs it will grow, develop and function on a level that you need and desire.

Look at a plant for instance, it needs specific elements to grow and bloom as do we.

So where did things go wrong?
Well as I mentioned before there are many influential factors in the mix but let's look at history.

When we were hunter gatherers we would live off what we could find and hunt, so these were the foundations of diet and served to fuel the body and enable it to function at a level that would allow us to do the daily tasks of hunting and gathering.

The tasks of early people were also done in the natural sunlight which is also a crucial factor of wellbeing.

All elements of this diet were natural and came from the earth. There were no processing methods that tampered with the food, it was as it was.

As the human race evolved man gained knowledge about food and experimented through time with combinations of herbs, spices and so on.

Then came the advent of agriculture and people went to town on creating new, exciting foods that tasted different and could be made more abundant to the masses.

Things such as breads and grains were widely utilised throughout the modern world as a source of convenience.

This swept the continent and more experimentation was prevalent.

The next stage was to preserve produced products so they lasted longer and longer.

Then as we skip to a more modern era creams and sauces were applied to amplify taste and enjoyment.

The above examples are from a time past so let's come to how these additions and techniques have changed modern foods.

In the search for abundant and tasty foods, we went 'nuts' and created product after product on a mass scale to supply the demand of the public.

These products comprised of different elements and were made up of so many different ingredients.

If you go to your local supermarket and pick up a product you may notice so many names that you don't quite understand.

Here is an example:

- **Brown Sugar**
- **Cane Crystals**
- **Cane Sugar**
- **Corn sweetener**
- **Corn syrup, or corn syrup solids**
- **Dehydrated Cane Juice**
- **Dextrin**
- **Dextrose**
- **Evaporated Cane Juice**
- **Glucose**
- **Honey**

- **Lactose**
- **Maltodextrin**
- **Malt syrup**
- **Maltose**
- **Maple syrup**
- **Molasses**
- **Palm Sugar**
- **Raw sugar**
- **Rice Syrup**
- **Saccharose**
- **Sucrose**
- **Xylose**

The previous list is an example of sugars that can be found in specific products.

Now the clients I have asked about these names didn't recognise 80% of them and wouldn't even read the labels to check what they were ingesting.

So all of the experimentation through time has created a multitude of elements that many people simply overlook and don't quite understand.

This is where we have gone wrong with our lack of knowledge as to what we are putting into our bodies.

Our bodies will work better if they are given the best materials we can provide to assist in correct function.

Through experience of eating and research I have learnt that a basic diet providing the key factors will heal you from inside out.

To re-educate ourselves in good nutrition is to give us the best chance of thriving naturally and resetting our bodies to a healthy state, free of depression and anxiety that are influenced by our diet.

We need to evaluate our current dietary habits and consumption so we can create new habits that will make our bodies function better.

By taking a look at ourselves and being brutally honest we can do a 360 degree turn and create a marvellous life.

So you're sat there saying 'Oh yeah whatever'

Let's look into what food can do for us to create this state of wellness.

BALANCE THE SCALES IN YOUR FAVOUR

FOOD AND ITS FUNCTIONS

I have, as mentioned, used food in the past as a comfort to hide away from my problems and give me momentary pleasure and also as a tool to lose weight and hopefully gain a better response from society and family.

You can have different relationships with food and it can serve the purpose that you give it.

For me, I used it as a tool and at first that tool was comfort.

Being bullied as a child I took solace in the simple joys of food, they comforted me in times of panic and crisis.

But it only fuelled the problem of being overweight unhealthy, de-motivated and energy-less.

The function for me was comfort, as in my mind it was there for me no matter what.

After years of pain and torture I then decided it was time to change and lose the weight.

So I did just that and lost more than what I planned and all my muscles were degenerated and small and I felt weak.

I then had comments and bullying from people who said I was too skinny; I felt I couldn't win and please anyone.

Then the depression, anxiety and pure 'O' came along which plagued me for many years until again I decided, 'enough was enough'.

I found diet had done so much to transform me so why couldn't it heal me from these debilitating conditions.

After much evaluation and countless days, weeks and months, I had come up with solutions I could implement to break free from my conditions and diet was a vital element.

If you want to know more of what I did I recommend you read my other book,

'There and Back The Dark Journey': The Way Back From Anxiety, Depression & Pure 'O'

You can find it on Amazon and other online outlets.

But this book is about diet and how it is a key factor in your recovery.

After I implemented specific dietary habits and changed my food consumption I noticed I had more energy and stamina to get the edge over my conditions.

When you are un-well you will literally do anything to find a guiding light to wellness and I have been 'through the mill' and back, but have found the light - you can too so keep with me here.

When I got well I could see that food should be respected as it gives the energy to live life at whatever level you choose.

It all comes down to the choices you make.

These choices have direct implications on your day to day life.

I chose to use food to help my mind and body function better and created a healthy relationship with food.

Food, as I say, serves you and you should optimise it to optimise your life.

Let me just give examples of how food can change your life, mind and body.

An athlete needs food to fuel their pursuits, re-generate energy and bodily tissues so they can recover quicker and perform at the highest level possible.

Someone who is morbidly obese uses food to lower their body mass which then has implications on their whole body and they are able to move more freely and live a more functional life.

They are able to be more independent and don't have to rely on others.

Their bones decompress and their organs are running at optimal levels instead of overdrive all the time.

Fat on the organs stops accumulating, creating better function and their chances of suffering from certain diseases decreases dramatically

The benefits of using food correctly are virtually endless.

Now you're thinking,' So what's it got to do with my condition and making me feel better?'

Well, when we give the body the building materials it needs to function optimally, we function on a higher level too.

So here is my example of the original guinea pig, 'me'.

I overhauled my diet to produce wellness and I did this in multiple ways and considered what implications certain foods had on the body.

These methods are not just utilised by me though, they have worked and continue to do so on my clients we have had some marvellous results.

But back to me......

First, I used the tool of evaluation and this took a lot when I was in the pits of despair, but knowing that wellness was my goal I was prepared to do anything.

Looking at my current lifestyle and dietary habits I noticed that I was not giving myself enough raw materials to function correctly.

EVALUATION is what you must do so I suggest you get a note pad and pen to write down your current food intake - don't worry about calories etc., at this point; all you need to know is what you are consuming.

Do this for a couple of weeks then take a look at the foods.

We can now implement the vital elements needed to bring about change.

HEAL YOURSELF INTERNALLY AND THE EXTERNAL WILL SOON FOLLOW

While you are evaluating, let's gain some knowledge of why food is of paramount importance to you gaining a restored, fully functioning system that makes you feel happy and free from your condition.

BUILD BACK YOUR HEALTH AND WELLBEING

KNOWLEDGE TIME

HERE WE GO.......

I don't want to go too technical here to confuse you, so we shall keep things simple.

The body is a complex machine capable of magnificent feats and to accomplish all of this the processes it undertakes require the correct building blocks to keep things up and running.

The body and mind are not separate and are linked with intricate systems that even with the research and knowledge of today we don't fully 100% understand.

There are pathways in the nervous system that operate to produce a specific function to make you do what you do day in and day out.

So if we don't provide the materials for these systems we get a fuse blown and things don't operate quite so smoothly.

We need good nutrition to help build and maintain optimum function and for the systems such as the brain to operate and produce the right chemicals/hormones for us to feel good.

Depression and anxiety take hold as the senses become on high alert and the building blocks we give the body are stolen and burnt away due to the state of constant fear, panic and crisis.

This knocks us out of 'whack' and our diets suffer and we don't provide the nutrients required in order to overcome this and restore normality.

Systems begin to suffer and the right balance of hormones and chemicals in the brain malfunction.

Let's take an example.

As you become depressed, anxious or down, Serotonin (neurotransmitter/feel good chemical) is one of the more widely recognised words especially as anxiety and depression cases rise.

We need a good balance of Serotonin to supply ourselves with the feel good factor - it is synthesized from the amino acid Tryptophan.

Serotonin makes us feel good and this is why when you go to the doctors regarding your condition they may mention anti depressants or SSRIs

S - Selective
S - **Serotonin**
R - Reuptake
I - Inhibitors

As you can see, I emphasised the word Serotonin as this is the element that is used to help the anti-depressant have an effect and make you feel good.

Research shows that reduced Serotonin can make you feel low, down, depressed and anxious.

It is the chemical that makes us feel good.

So we need to put all the keystones together and utilise nutrition effectively and build up our Serotonin.

HOW??

Well because Tryptophan synthesises Serotonin we need to incorporate foods that contain it such as:

- Turkey
- Egg white
- Salmon
- Crab
- Seaweed
- Pumpkin Seeds
- Squash Seeds
- Chicken

These are a few examples.
So here we see an example of how Serotonin levels can effect your body.

Try the following recipes:

Salmon Scrambled egg & Whole wheat Bagel

Ingredients:

- 3 Eggs (use 1 whole egg and 2 whites)
- Salmon (oven cooked)
- Whole wheat bagel
- Pepper (to taste)

Simple and quick.

All you need to do is scramble the eggs then cook your salmon, mash together and put on your bagel with a pinch of pepper to taste.

Pumpkin Seed Salad

Ingredients:

- Pumpkin seeds (small cupped hand full)
- 2 large lettuce leafs
- Chopped pepper
- Sweet corn

- Chicken/Turkey or Crab (shredded)
- Beetroot
- Onion
- 1 Boiled egg
- Drizzle of extra virgin olive oil
- Cucumber
- Tomato
- Feta cheese

I usually make a large salad and save some in the refrigerator for another time,

For this salad you simply combine all the given ingredients then toss the salad and you have a healthy meal.

Let's explore more options that will aid you in your quest to restoring a balanced system.

THE BODY IS A COMPLEX MACHINE JUST LIKE A CAR AND YOU NEED TO FILL A CAR WITH THE RIGHT FLUIDS, OILS ETC., TO RUN IT PROPERLY AND IT'S THE SAME WITH THE BODY & YOUR NUTRITION, ESPECIALLY IF YOU WANT TO REACH YOUR POTENTIAL

SHOW ME THE LIGHT

SAY WHAT?

The next subject I want to talk about is obtaining precious vitamin D levels in the body.

When many people become anxious or depressed they often retreat indoors and don't give it a second thought as situations often become so overwhelming.

I know when I first evaluated myself I noted that I would spend 90 % if not more of my time hidden away in my room crying.

This was a regular thing, but once I had realised this in my evaluation I noticed I was depriving my body of the richest source of vitamin D.

I was not getting the vitamin from the sun and therefore my system was becoming even more imbalanced.

More and more research is showing that vitamin D levels are linked with low mood and depression.

Now you say 'why?'

Well, vitamin D is absorbed by the body through sunlight and used to produce a stable balance.

You may have heard of SAD

S - **Seasonal**

A - **Affective**

D - **Disorder**

As you can see, it's in the name.

Basically the season affects your mood as sunlight is not as prevalent in the winter as it is in the summer therefore it affects the natural levels of vitamin D in the body.

You will notice in colder countries where the sun is scarce that there is a higher percentage of SAD cases compared to warmer climates.

You're saying, 'Light? I can't eat that' - well 'no' but it should be part of your daily routine and you can also obtain sources from foods such as:

- Salmon - nice done in the oven with a drizzle of lemon.
- Trout
- Tuna - good on a sandwitch or in a salad and it is rich in protein too!!!
- Egg yolks - fantastic scrambled with toast.
- Offal

Try incorporating the foods above into your diet.

If you are concerned about your vitamin D levels consult your doctor and he/she will usually send you for a blood test.

Also you can but special SAD lights which you utilise to help gain the balance back.

I have one at the side of my bed and usually use it in the winter months but I get outside as much as I possibly can.

It's good to schedule outdoor time into your day so that your vitamin D intake is being constantly topped up.

AS PART OF YOUR DAILY DIET UTILISE OUTDOOR TIME TO OBTAIN PRECIOUS VITAMIN D

OMEGA 3

This is more than often a scary subject when I discuss it with my clients.

When I mention the word 'fat' I see a puzzled look cross their faces as there has been so much debate over fats in the diet over the years.

But the brain is made up of nearly 60% fat.

Why is this so important?

The omega 6 helps promote inflammation in the body which is great when you are hurt, as this is the body's natural response to help heal itself, but when an abundance of omega 6 is introduced this system goes into overdrive and can affect the functioning of the brain.

This we don't want!!!

We need a better balance of the omegas and the best way is to INCREASE omega 3's (which help **Serotonin** function) and decrease omega 6's.

You can do this through supplementation - ask for more information at your local health store, do a little research you will find this has helped many people, me included.

I chose to supplement and take mine every morning with a glass of water.

But you can also increase your omega 3s through diet by consuming foods such as:

- Flaxseed - can be sprinkled on salads/cereals/porridge
- Walnuts - good as a quick snack or can be put on salads - I know my mother loves a few walnuts on her salad and I do too.
- Salmon
- Tofu - great choice for vegetarians and is rich in protein.

- Sardines - I like to make a tomatoe sauce to go with sardines and have them on a bagel to give a really nice texture.
- Mussels
- Chia Seeds

IF YOU WANT CHANGE THERE IS ONLY YOU WHO HAS THE ABILITY TO MAKE IT HAPPEN

PEP YOURSELF UP BY GETTING YOUR B VITAMINS

The reason I included the B vitamins is because they are widely utilised throughout the body.

Let's take a look:

Thiamine aka vitamin B1

This is utilised by the body to convert glucose into energy, so low levels will affect our energy levels and alertness by making us feel tired.

I know that in an anxious/depressed state energy drains very quickly and robs the body/ mind of its sharpness, so that's why we need to combat this through nutrition.

Here are some good sources of B1:

- Sunflower seeds
- Pork
- Macadamia nuts

- Asparagus - I love these grilled with a small sprinkle of sea salt.
- Butternut Squash - you can add this to soups or roast in the oven. Also if you are doing mash potatoes try sweet potato and Butternut squash mashed together.

Next, Niacin aka vitamin B3

B3 has gained much popularity over the years and I first heard about it from a documentary and then through research and my nutrition qualification.

The more I learnt, the more willing I was to incorporate it into my diet as there have also been documented cases of it assisting to aid sufferers of depression/anxiety.

Here are a few examples:

- Portobello mushrooms

- Chicken - salads/casseroles/sandwitches/vegtables
- Pork
- Prawns - good for seafood salads/sandwitches
- Salmon
- Tuna
- Avocado - I always liked Avocado with Feta cheese and sun blushed tomatoes plus a side salad.

Next Pantothenic Acid aka B5
This helps with memory and the ability to retain/learn information which when depressed/anxious is key to obtaining the tools necessary for recovery.

Example foods:

- Eggs - scrambled or poached are my favourite options.
- Trout - great cooked with lemon or orange slices on top in the oven.
- Mushrooms - I love mushrooms and they can be stuffed with feta cheese

or put into soups which are my favorite two options.
- Avocado
- Pork
- Sunflower seeds - as a quick snack or add to your salads.
- Sweet potato - baking them or peel them and roast them in the oven with a drizzle of extra virgin olive oil - my dad loves it when I cook these.

<u>B6 aka Pyridoxine</u>

Often a favourite in the exercise/bodybuilding community, B6 aids in protein metabolism.

But it also helps to convert **Tryptophan** into **Serotonin** which is vital to the feel good factor and a happy mood as we discussed earlier.

Example foods:

- Spinach - I try to add spinach as much as I can. Use it in salads or

on sandwiches. You can incorporate it into stif fry too.
- Pistachio nuts - again a quick snack or you can add to salads
- Lentils - Fantastic in soups I love to incorporate lentils with home made curry.
- Kale - this is awesome you can add it to stir fry or on homemade burgers
- Bananas - One of my most recent recipes for bannanas is:

Get one banana and mash it up as finely as possible then whisk up 1 whole egg and two whites.

Next add the banana and eggs together and mix as much as possible then sprinkle on some cinnamon.

(I know sounds a bit crazy but I love em)

Then get your frying pan out and put some coconut oil in and wait for it to melt.

Then add your mixture and make it into a pancake. Put on your plate when its finished add a few Blueberries and enjoy mmmmmmm :)

As you can see from the B vitamin groups they do the body good and help it to function at a more efficient level which is what we require when tackling anxiety/depression and the tasks of daily life.

GIVE YOUR BODY THE TOOLS IT NEEDS TO GET WELL AND YOU'RE ON YOUR WAY TO BEING WELL AGAIN!!!

Glutamine

Another favourite of the bodybuilding community for its effects on the ability to maintain lean muscle mass and aid in recovery.

Glutamine has been used to also combat things such as:

- Stress
- Depression
- Low mood
- Enhanced performance
- Mental alertness
- Increased energy output

Glutamine can really help you to recover and rebuild so it is vital we gain this amino acid through either supplementation or diet.

Examples:

- Eggs
- Beef

- Cottage cheese - awesome in salads or as a quick snack which provides a good hit of protein too.
- Lentils
- Peas
- Beans

Tryptophan

We mentioned this before, so you know how vital it is to keep levels topped up.

Iron

Low levels of iron can make you become anaemic and this brings fatigue and can cause you to feel energy-less and depressed.

So it's best to top up your levels by eating iron rich foods.

- Spinach
- Liver
- Vegetables - can be eaten cooked or raw whichever you prefer.

Magnesium

Magnesium has a reputation of having a calming effect and also plays a vital role in almost every part of the body. You can get yours by eating:

- Dark, leafy greens
- Cashew nuts
- Sunflower seeds
- Salmon

Multi-vitamin

I take a multi-vitamin to cover the bases - on the next page a word on supplements.

TO BRING CHANGE YOU MUST USE ACTION

SUPPLEMENTATION

Before you do anything, discuss it with your G.P to make sure you have the best help possible.

I always say though that food should be your first port of call when trying to get the vital elements in place.

Supplements are as always in addition to the diet, to supplement a lack of nutrients that you haven't quite covered in your diet.

So as a kick start I used supplements at the beginning and as my mood improved I incorporated more foods and a good variety too.

I still have supplements too but have a fantastically nutrient dense diet now which keeps me happy and healthy and gives my body what it needs to remain balanced.

There are a wealth of supplements out there that can really help jump start your approach to getting better.

BUT

There are the drawbacks too.

Make sure that you get the best quality and do a little research and always buy from a trusted retailer.

Always be on your guard against people trying to sell you something that is displayed as one thing but unknown to you and is another.

I get my supplements through a well known retailer with certified products - make sure you buy the best possible that suits your budget.

I CAN PROVIDE YOU WITH THE KNOWLEDGE AND TOOLS BUT IT'S UP TO YOU TO IMPLEMENT THEM

STIMULATION

We have gone through a handful of helpful vitamins, so now a word on stimulants.

Over the last ten years stimulant drinks have been on the rise and seen as the thing to drink, especially amongst teenagers and young adults.

There are many people who drink too much caffeine which causes their nervous system to be like a phone on vibrate.

These stimulants stimulate the body by giving quick bursts of energy making you feel like you could jump in the air and run, run, run.

Now I know research has show that ergogenic aids are used by people who wish to enhance their performance in a specific physical activity which is all well and good.

But this book is for people who want to recover from anxiety/depression/pure 'O' so we don't require nervous energy that could force the body to go into an all-out panic attack.

This is exactly what we do not want, so I suggest (as I did) you lower your caffeine levels so that your nervous system doesn't get shaky and upset so as to stimulate an episode of panic.

Replace your intake with caffeine free drinks such as:

- Water
- Caffeine free tea
- Flavoured water

GAIN THE ADVANTAGE OVER YOUR CURRENT CONDITION & RECLAIM YOUR LIFE BACK

STABILITY

When I evaluated myself I could see that there was no consistency or stability in my entire diet.

I would simply reach for what was there and retreat to my safety zone, my darkened room.

The foods I would eat were very convenient and cheap sources of not very nutritious foods and so my body had no stability.

I would often use food as a comfort so that meant to me chocolate which was eaten in larger quantities which would provoke blood sugar spikes.

Not a very helpful thing when you want to be calm but I had to look back, reflect and change what was out of balance.

So I noticed the spikes only assisted in making me panic and inducing an all out attack on my system.

If I wanted stability to restore my mind I needed to stabilise my blood sugar levels to retain a constant flow of energy instead of highs and lows.

That's when I took action and went back to my training and devised a diet that would stabilise my blood sugars.

I needed to choose foods that would help maintain energy and not give me nervous levels throughout the day.

I chose to ditch the sugary/overly processed junk foods and replace them with vitamin/mineral rich foods.

OUT

- Chocolates
- Crisps
- Buns
- Cakes
- Pastries
- White flour products
- Pop
- Coffee

IN

- Vegetables
- Small portions of fruit
- Whole grains
- Water, water and more water
- Salads
- Fish
- Lean meat
- Small helpings of nuts
- Soy
- seeds

This was a drastic change but I can't tell you how much of a difference it made to my energy and likelihood of having a panic attack.

I was giving my body what it needed to thrive and heal inside out.

Now nutrition is one tool you can utilise to help yourself gain wellness and a restored balance throughout the mind and body.

I CAN DO IT - SO CAN YOU

ALL ABOUT THE BALANCE

It really is all about balancing the scales in your favour.

Diet is a crucial component in any pursuit, even in the pursuit of a depression/anxiety/pure 'O' free life.

You have to look at the evidence of what food does to the body.

There are so many processes undertaken by your body on a day to day basis that if I were to describe them all you would still be reading the book in two years time!!!

From muscle growth to the production of Serotonin, the body has a multitude of processes to go through to enable it to operate optimally.

So it makes sense that we should provide it with the tools and building materials to do just that, day in day out.

Now I'm not telling you to deprive yourself forever, but assist yourself back to good health and then you can afford to treat yourself occasionally.

So remember, the first step is **evaluation** and the next is **implementation**.

You have to look at your diet and make decisions from your evaluation of where you can change things for the better.

Start slowly and make the following basic changes to your diet:

- Drink more water - this will keep the body regulated and help to prevent dehydration.
- Reduce sugary foods - things that spike your blood sugar quickly could make you panic, so reduce your junk food such as sweets or chocolate.
- Lower caffeine intake - this will lower your nervous energy levels which could make you panic.

- Eat small nutritious meals - eat regular small meals to keep your body satisfied and stable throughout the day.
- Try herbal teas - herbal teas can have a soothing effect which again will help you to remain calm.
- Get plenty of vegetables - by getting your veggies you are filling your body with fibre and vitamins/minerals.

The above list is a base where you should start from.

Don't over complicate things and start with small simple changes that you implement over time.

IT TAKES TIME BUT YOU WILL GET THERE

BE PREPARED

You need to do some prep if you want to be consistent with your nutrition and create positive habits and change in your life.

Here are some tips for you to use:

- Keep a diary so you can see what foods you currently consume and what foods you want to incorporate.
- Have a recipe sheet on hand so that you don't grow bored.
- Get a BPA free bottle so you have water handy all day long.
- Stock up on herbs and spices so you can give your foods great flavour.
- Get a family member or friend to help you on your journey and support each other.
- Buy organic whenever possible so you are giving your body the best quality possible.
- Make a habit of reading food labels
- Use BPA free tubs to store pre prepared foods.

FINAL WORDS

I want to thank you for buying this material and taking time to focus on the most important person YOU.

I am constantly doing what I can, when I can, to help as many people possible.

So please come and join me on Facebook simply type:

Self Help/Motivation Books & Audio

I wish you all the best and continued success in your journey to wellness.

FEEL GOOD ABOUT THE STEPS YOU ARE TAKING TO BE WELL - Please visit:

www.hungry4fitness.blogspot.com

NOTES:

www.ingramcontent.com/pod-product-compliance
Lightning Source LLC
Chambersburg PA
CBHW020930180526
45163CB00007B/2964